Flossopher says:

"I floss and brush, therefore I am happy."

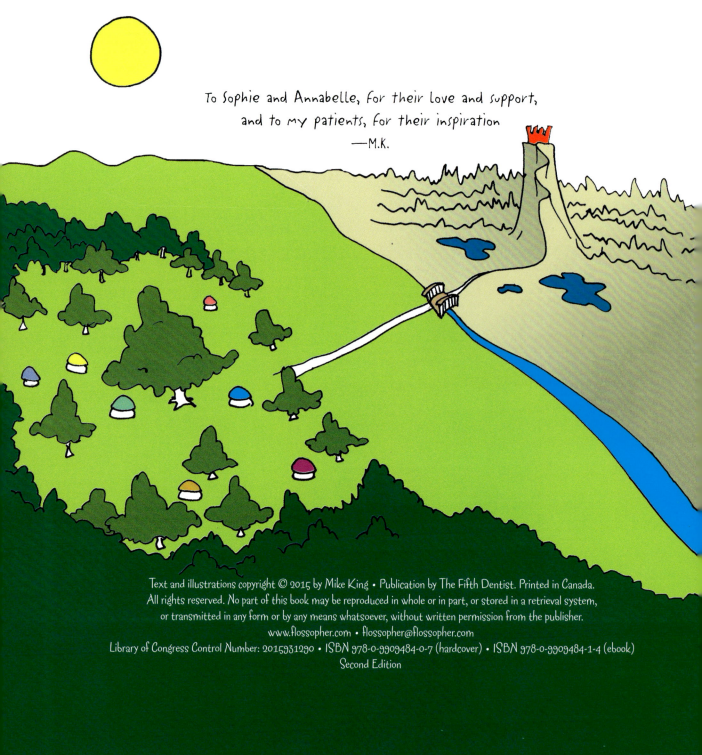

Flossopher and the Brushing Trees
An Adventure for Young Tooth Brushers

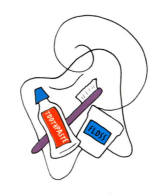

By "Dr. Mike" King
Illustrations by Rick Ellis

Publication by The Fifth Dentist

This is Flossopher.

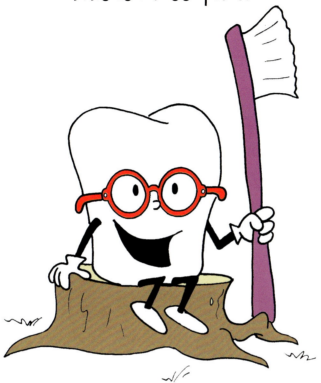

He lives in the Brite Forest and knows everything there is to know about taking care of teeth.

His job is to make sure that everyone who lives in the Brite Forest keeps their teeth clean and sparkly.

"You have to brush your teeth at least twice a day: after breakfast and before going to bed," Flossopher tells his friends.

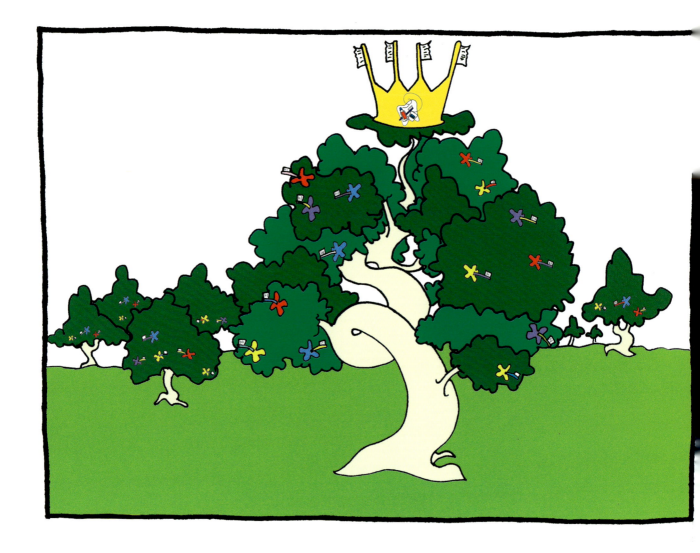

These are the Brushing Trees. They are very special, magical trees. They grow toothbrushes. And they grow only in the Brite Forest.

The biggest of the Brushing Trees is Sparkla. She's the mother of all Brushing Trees and the most magical of them all. Without the magic from her Brush Crown, none of the other Brushing Trees would be able to grow brushes.

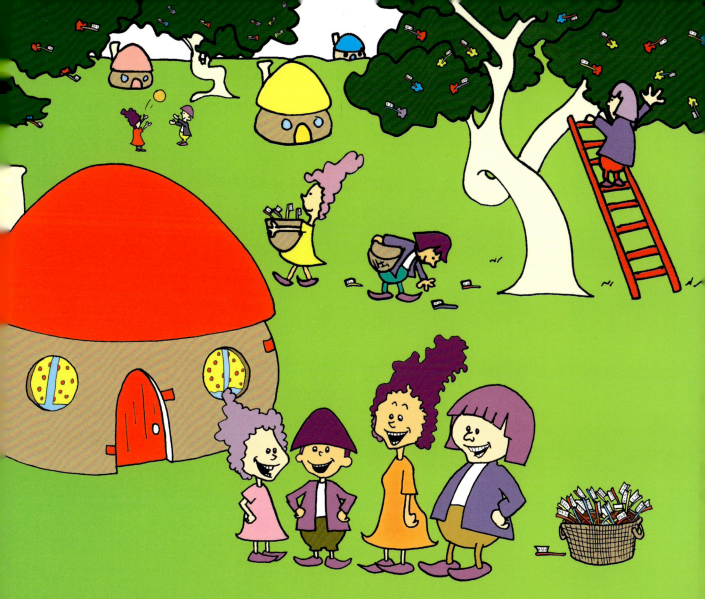

These are Flossopher's friends and helpers—the Brushers. They are small, but not too small. They have purple hair, but not too purple. Their job is very important. They pick the toothbrushes from the Brushing Trees so that everyone else in the Brite Forest can have their own toothbrush.

Far away is the land called Durt, where the evil Cavidorg lives high atop Mount Yuk.

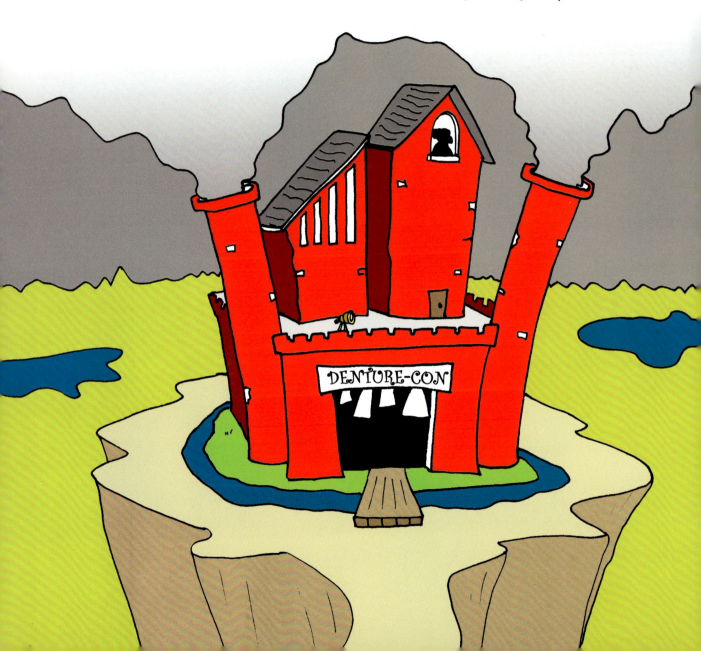

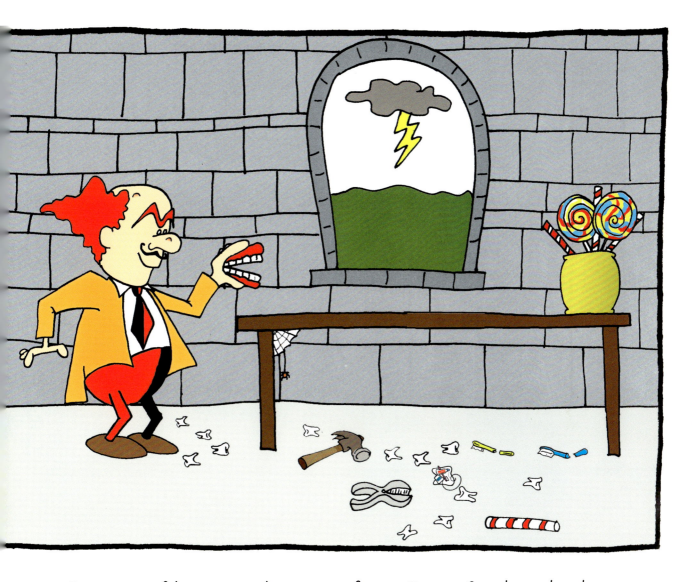

Cavidorg loves fake plastic teeth and owns a factory, Denture-Con, that makes them. Cavidorg hates toothbrushes that keep real teeth clean, so he's always plotting ways to keep Flossopher and his friends from brushing their teeth. That way, everyone's teeth will rot and fall out. Then Denture-Con will be able to sell even more fake teeth to the world.

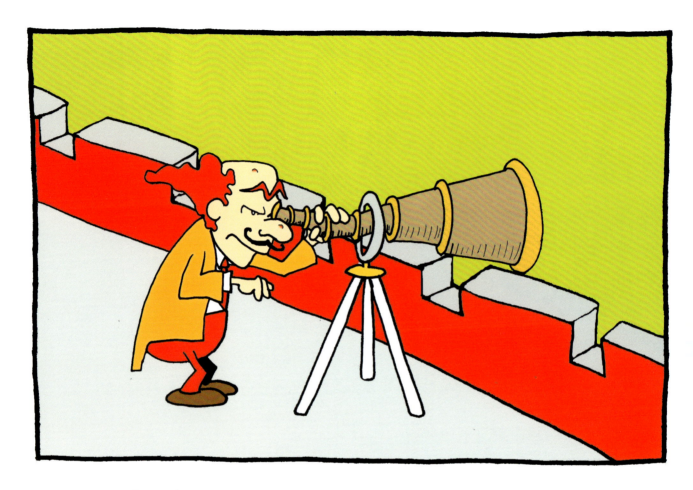

From his lookout tower on Mount Yuk, Cavidorg keeps watch. When someone in the Brite Forest doesn't brush their teeth, a dark cloud forms in the sky. That's bad for the forest, but good for Cavidorg. The more clouds there are above the Brite Forest, the darker it will become. If it gets dark enough, Cavidorg can send in his army of dirty, rotten Cavity Bugs to steal Sparkla's Brush Crown. Then none of the Brushing Trees will grow toothbrushes, and no one will be able to brush. Denture-Con will be busy forever!

Cavidorg sees a dark cloud forming above the Brite Forest. He rubs his hands together and laughs an evil laugh.

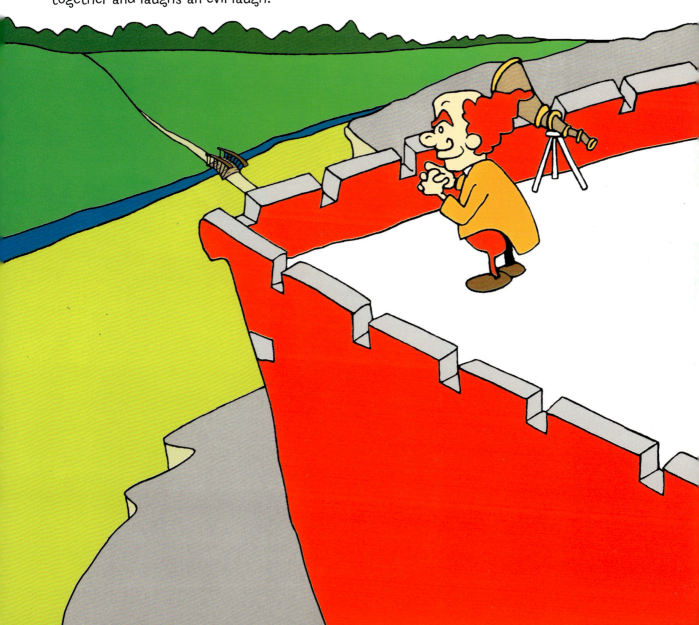

"Come here, Shugrot! Get over here, Dirtlum!" Cavidorg summons his sneakiest Cavity Bugs and explains his twisted plot to them.

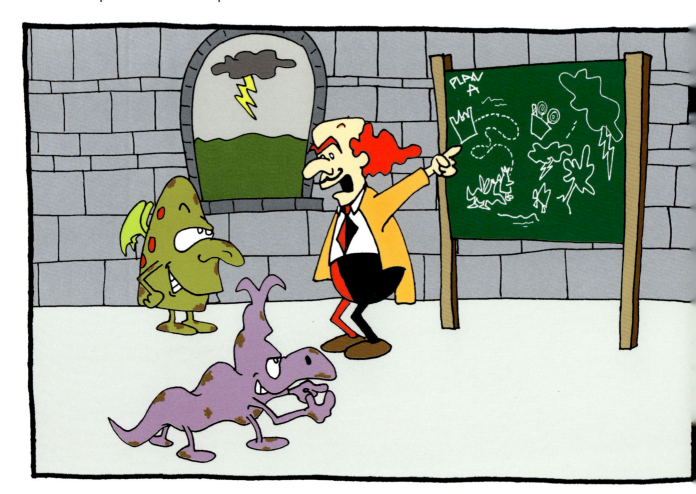

The dirty, rotten Cavity Bugs love the plan.

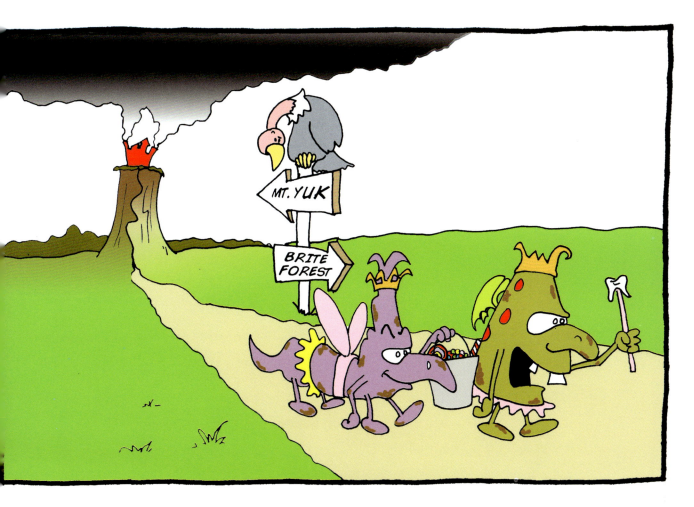

They get dressed up as tooth fairies and set off for the Brite Forest in disguise.

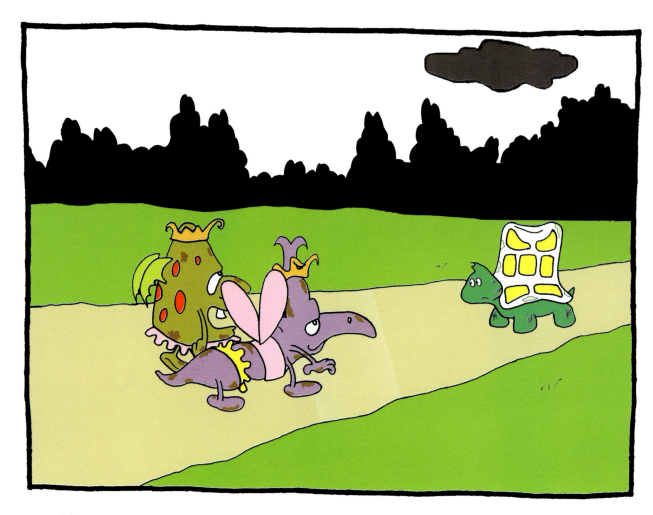

Shugrot and Dirtlum soon find Toothyl Turtle under the dark cloud. She has lost her toothbrush and hasn't brushed her teeth in two whole days.

"Wow!" says Toothyl. "Could it be? Tooth fairies? *Two* tooth fairies?"

"It's your lucky day," says Dirtlum. "We're here because you've been so good at not (heh-heh) brushing. We came to give you—"

"Yummy candy!" interrupts Shugrot. "Mmm. Go ahead, eat it. Eat it ALL!"

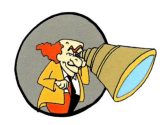

"You mean all of this is for me?" asks Toothyl. "It looks so good. Yumm!"

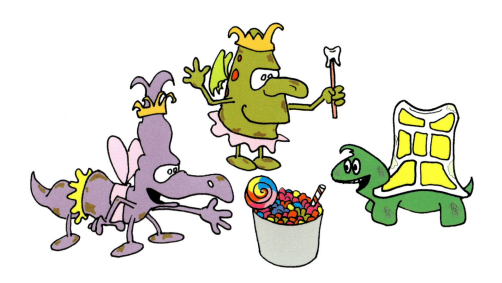

"But wait." She remembers what Flossopher has told her. "Aren't eating candy and not brushing bad for my teeth?"

"This is special candy," says Dirtlum. "You won't ever have to brush again."

"Heh, heh, heh," snickers Cavidorg as he watches from Mount Yuk and sees how well his plan is working. "Of course she won't ever have to brush again. She won't have any teeth left to brush!"

"Trust us," says Shugrot. "We're tooth fairies."

Toothyl hesitates, then reaches for the candy. "Well, okay," she says.

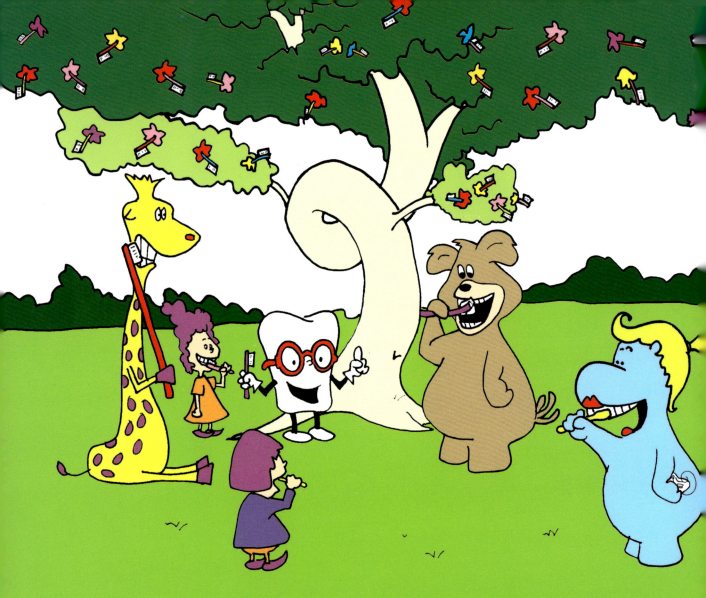

Meanwhile, Flossopher is conducting a brushing class under Sparkla's branches. "Make sure you brush all the way in the back of your mouth. The back teeth are the hardest to keep clean," he tells his friends.

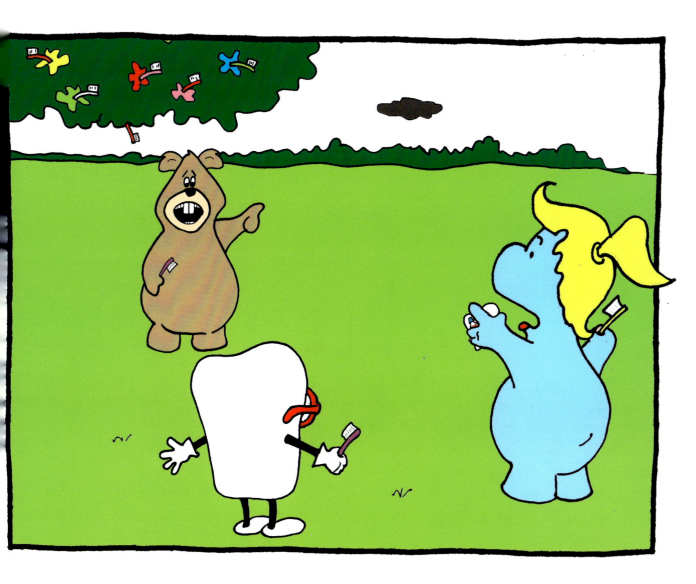

"Flossopher, look!" Bucky Bear points. "There's a cloud over the Brite Forest!"
"Quick! Someone hasn't brushed and needs your help!" says Lippo Hippo.
"Yikes!" says Flossopher. "I'll grab my special toothbrush and be on my way!"

Flossopher gets there just in the nick of time!

"Stop, Toothyl!" he yells. "Don't eat that candy!"

Then he turns to the Cavity Bugs. "Get away from her, Shugrot and Dirtlum! I'll give you a brushing you'll never forget!"

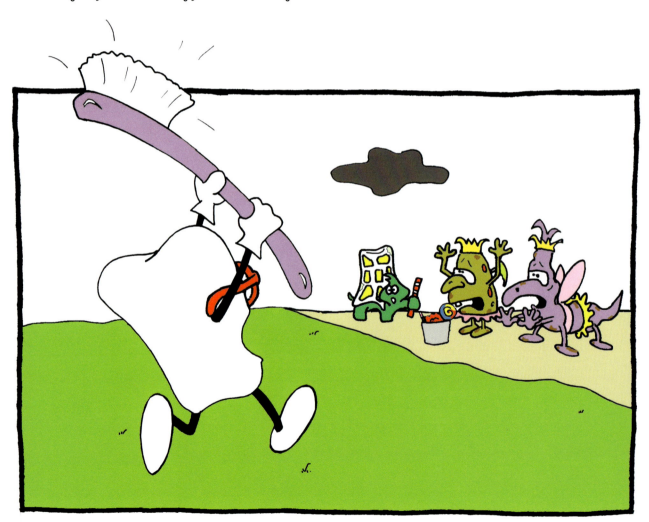

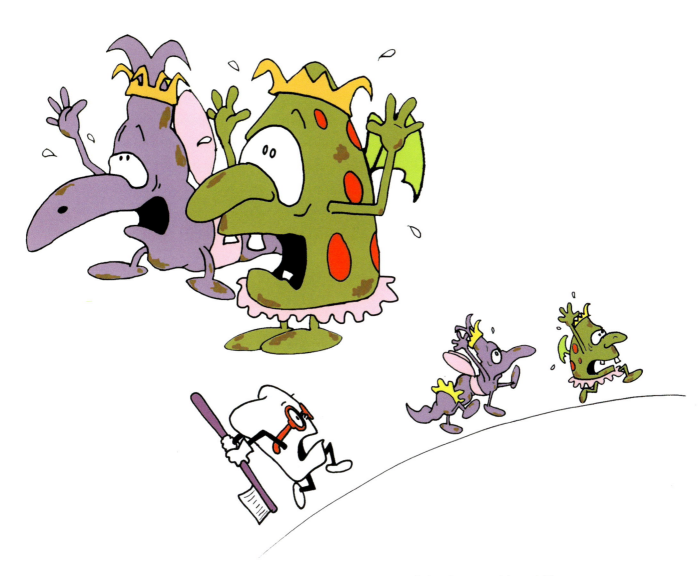

"Run!!" yell Shugrot and Dirtlum. "It's Flossopher with his big toothbrush!"
Shugrot and Dirtlum run away. If Flossopher brushes them, they'll lose their dirt and grime, and they'll never be allowed back on Mount Yuk.

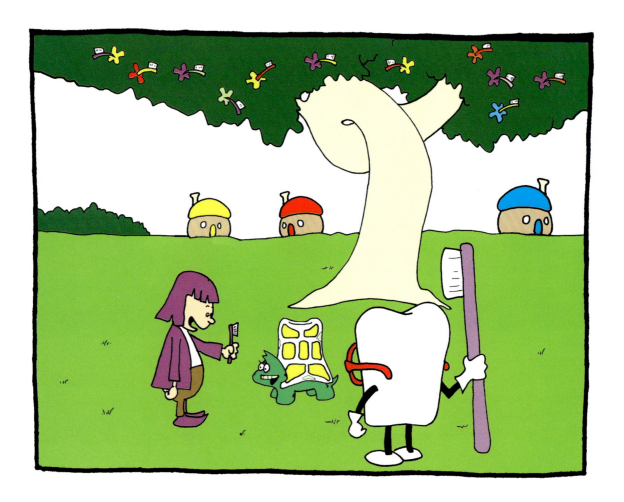

"Whew!" says Flossopher. "That was close! Toothyl, are you all right? You look a little dirty. Where is your toothbrush?"

Toothyl looks at the ground, embarrassed. "I lost it . . . um, two days ago," she says.

"Uh-oh! Quick, we'd better get you a new one."

A Brusher steps forward and hands Toothyl a brush. "Here you go. I picked this one right off the branches of Sparkla herself. And now it's yours."

"Thank you!" says Toothyl. She brushes long and carefully.

"I'm clean again!" she says happily.

Flossopher says, "You look marvelous! Now, try not to lose your toothbrush again. But if you do, let me know right away. Remember, Cavidorg is always watching."

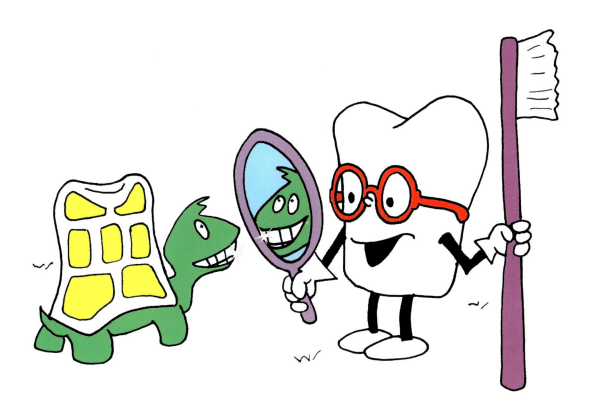

Back on Mount Yuk, Cavidorg is furious. "What?! No more clouds over the Brite Forest?" he yells. "Aughh!!"

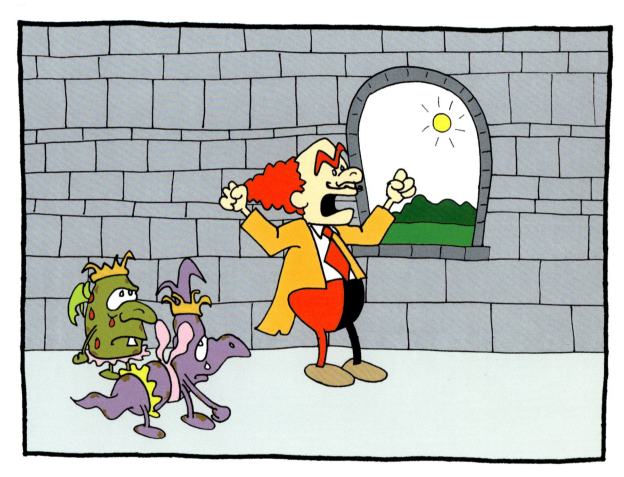

"You may have won this time, Flossopher. But mark my words, one day the Brite Forest will be mine!!"

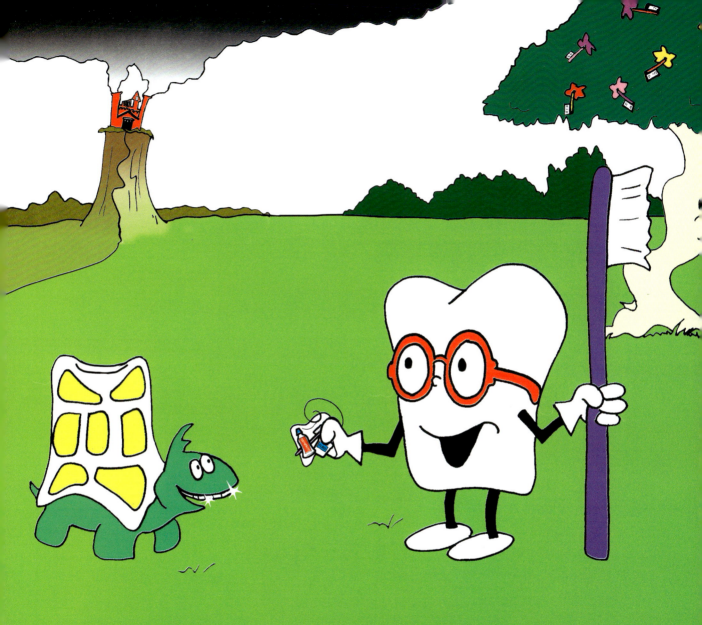

From far away, Flossopher hears him and replies, "Not if we brush twice a day, eat healthy foods, and floss! But that's a story for another day!"

Flossopher's Instructions for Brushing

1| Put a pea-sized amount of toothpaste on a soft-bristle toothbrush.

2| Hold the brush at an angle to your teeth so that the bristles point toward your gums.

 3| Brush each tooth by moving the toothbrush in small circles.

4| Brush all the surfaces of your teeth: Outside. Inside.

Tops of bottom teeth. Bottoms of top teeth. Don't forget the very back teeth.

 5| When you're finished brushing, rinse, swish, and spit.

Flossopher says, "Remember, keep Cavidorg away! Brush twice a day!"

This is a tooth-care kit. Seven kits (including this one) are shown in this book. Five are easy to find, but you have to look really carefully to find the other two. Can you find them all?